Super Easy Healthy Heart Cookbook For Beginners

Effortless and Nutritious: A Beginner's Guide to Easy, Healthy Cooking

Antonio D. Myers

Table of content

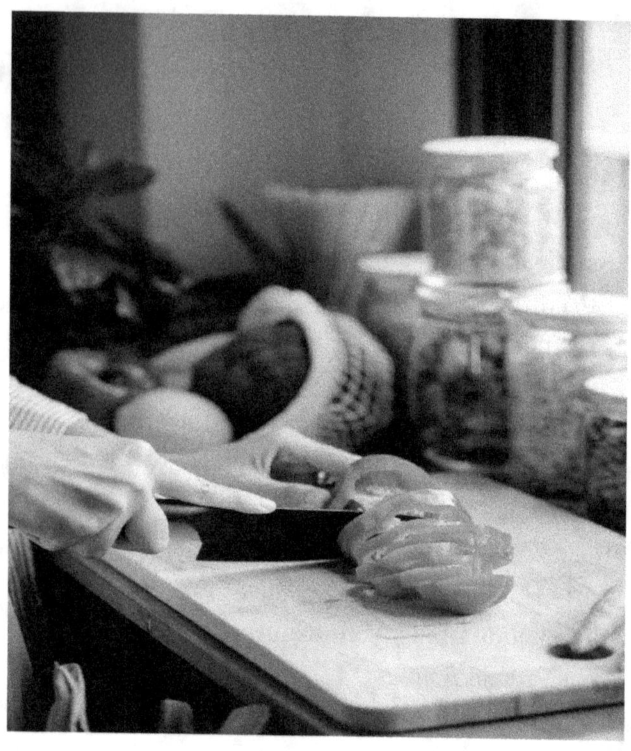

Introduction

Alice was a woman who lived in Brooksville, a busy city. Although Alice was well-known for her love of cooking, she hadn't been feeling well lately. She had little energy and was frequently tired. She chose to see her doctor since she was worried about her health Following a battery of examinations, the physician advised Alice that her cardiac condition required monitoring.

She was told to drastically alter her diet after receiving a high cholesterol diagnosis. Alice was feeling overwhelmed and went to her local bookstore where she found the "Healthy Heart Cookbook" as a source of help. Excited, Alice delved into the cookbook, discovering a treasure trove of heart-healthy recipes.

With renewed determination, she began experimenting in her kitchen, swapping out unhealthy ingredients for nutritious alternatives. Her culinary adventures led her to explore vibrant flavors and fresh ingredients she hadn't considered before.

As Alice embraced her newfound passion for heart-healthy cooking, she noticed remarkable changes in how she felt. Her energy levels soared, and the constant fatigue faded away. She felt lighter, both physically and emotionally, as she nourished her body with wholesome meals.

Word of Alice's transformation spread throughout the neighborhood, inspiring others to embark on their own journey to better health. Encouraged by her progress, Alice started hosting cooking workshops, sharing her knowledge and recipes with those eager to improve their heart health.

Months passed, and Alice's kitchen became a hub of activity and laughter, filled with the aroma of delicious, heart-healthy creations. Her cookbook became dog-eared and stained, a testament to her culinary adventures and the joy she found in taking care of her heart.
With each meal she prepared, Alice poured her heart and soul into her cooking, knowing that she was not only nourishing her body but also nurturing her spirit. And as she savored each bite, she felt grateful for the journey that had led her to rediscover the simple joy of good

food and good health.Greetings from the delectable world of heart-healthy cuisine! This beginner-friendly cookbook is a symphony of tastes designed to feed the body and the soul.

Every meal showcases healthful ingredients and straightforward methods, ranging from colorful salads to soothing soups and delectable main courses. Prepare to go on a culinary journey that will not only satisfy your palate but also promote heart health. One delectable dish at a time, let's celebrate the blessing of good health and the joy of cooking.

Chapter 1 Understanding Heart Health

Anatomy and Function: The heart is a muscular organ that uses the circulatory system to circulate blood throughout the body. A basic understanding of the heart's anatomy, including its chambers, valves, and arteries, is necessary to comprehend heart health.

Risk factors: A number of variables, such as smoking, high blood pressure, high cholesterol, diabetes, obesity, poor diet, inactivity, excessive alcohol consumption, and stress, can lead to heart disease. For heart health, it is crucial to identify these risk factors and take appropriate action.

Prevention: The best way to avoid heart disease is to have a heart-healthy lifestyle. This entails keeping a healthy weight, exercising frequently, abstaining from smoking and excessive alcohol use, managing stress, and eating a balanced diet full of fruits, vegetables, complete grains, and lean meats.

Evaluation and Prognosis: Monitoring heart health requires routine visits to a physician. Electrocardiograms (ECGs), blood pressure checks, cholesterol assessments, and other screening procedures can identify risk factors and early indicators of heart disease.

Recognizing Symptoms: Being aware of the warning signs and symptoms of cardiac issues, such as fatigue, dizziness, shortness of breath, chest discomfort, and irregular heartbeat, can help you get medical help when you need it.

Cardiovascular Diseases: Managing and avoiding various cardiovascular diseases, such as coronary artery disease, heart failure, arrhythmias, and heart valve abnormalities, requires an understanding of these conditions' causes, symptoms, risk factors, and available treatments.

Cardiovascular rehabilitation, medicine, angioplasty, bypass surgery, and, in certain situations, heart transplantation are among the possible treatment options for heart disease. Working closely with healthcare providers and being aware of these possibilities can help maximize results.

Effective management is essential for minimizing problems and maintaining heart health in people with chronic illnesses such high blood pressure, diabetes, or high cholesterol.

Campaigns for public awareness, educational programs, and other resources are essential for encouraging heart health and giving people the knowledge they need to make decisions regarding their cardiovascular health.

Innovation and Research: Heart disease is becoming better understood, prevented, diagnosed, and treated because of ongoing cardiology research and improvements. Both patients and healthcare providers may make educated decisions by keeping up with the most recent advancements.

Understanding anatomy, risk factors, prevention techniques, symptoms, diseases, available treatments, and continuing research are all important components of a thorough grasp of heart health. Through proactive prevention and treatment strategies and a focus on heart health, people can lower their risk of cardiovascular illnesses and lead healthier, more active lives.

Essential Ingredients and Kitchen Tools

It's essential to have the right tools and supplies while preparing heart-healthy dishes. Let's start with the parts:

Ingredients:

Whole Grains: Integrating whole grains like brown rice, quinoa, oats, and barley into your culinary repertoire not only adds a wholesome touch but also provides a plethora of fiber, vitamins, and minerals crucial for cardiovascular wellness. These grains, replete with low cholesterol and saturated fats, serve as the cornerstone of heart-friendly dishes.

Lean Proteins: Adopt a diet that includes skinless chicken, tofu, lentils, beans, fish (particularly omega-3 fatty acid-rich varieties like salmon, trout, and mackerel), and legumes. Acclaimed for providing vital nutrients without raising cholesterol, these protein powerhouses are low in saturated fat.

Good Fats: When making recipes, use foods like avocados, nuts (almonds, walnuts, and pistachios), seeds (chia and flax seeds), and olive oil as sources of good fats. When eaten in moderation, these lipid heroes—rich in monounsaturated and polyunsaturated fats—can support heart health by lowering the risk of heart disease and helping to regulate cholesterol.

Using a variety of vibrant fruits and vegetables, such as apples, berries, citrus fruits, bell peppers, tomatoes, and carrots, can enhance the color and vitality of your food preparation. Full of vitamins, minerals, and antioxidants, these plant-based wonders support heart health by lowering blood pressure and cholesterol levels and strengthening circulatory function.

Low-Sodium Options: Reduce your consumption of sodium, a major contributor to hypertension and cardiovascular diseases, by choosing low-sodium or no-salt-added canned products, sauces, and condiments. Increase taste without adding too much sodium by using herbs, spices, and citrus liquids as savory alternatives.

Kitchen Tools:

Precision Knives: Add these to your kitchen arsenal to be able to chop and slice fruits, veggies, and lean meats with ease. Sharp blades ensure uniform cuts that facilitate even cooking in addition to streamlining meal preparation.

Cutting Board: Make an investment in a sturdy cutting board made of plastic or wood, which will offer a steady surface for easily and precisely chopping ingredients. To reduce the possibility of cross-contamination and prioritize food safety, use separate boards for Steamer Basket: Use a steamer basket's versatility to perfectly prepare fish, veggies, and cereals without adding extra fat. Steam cooking encourages heart-healthy culinary pursuits by preserving the natural nutrients and flavors of ingredients. meats and produce.

Non-Stick Cookware: Embrace non-stick pots and pans to minimize oil usage during cooking, thereby reducing added fats and calories. Opt for cookware boasting ceramic or PTFE-free coatings to ensure safer culinary practices.

Measuring Cups and Spoons: Measure ingredients precisely with measuring cups and spoons to improve your cooking skills. Precise measurement-taking guarantees that heart-healthy recipes have the right amount of nutrients in the right proportions, opening the door to healthful cooking.

Oven Thermometer: Elevate your baking prowess with the aid of an oven thermometer, ensuring precise temperature control for flawlessly cooked meals. By safeguarding against undercooked or overcooked dishes, an oven thermometer not only enhances culinary outcomes but also bolsters food safety protocols.

Equipped with these necessary components and culinary implements, you're ready to set off on a gastronomic adventure full of heart-healthy treats that entice the palate and promote cardiovascular well-being.

Breakfast Delights

A heart-healthy breakfast can provide you with a satisfying start to the day. Imagine waking up to the aroma of hot, freshly cooked quinoa or oats simmering with a touch of cinnamon on top. Excellent providers of soluble fiber, which lowers cholesterol and promotes heart health by lowering the risk of cardiovascular disease, are these whole grains.

Imagine adding a colorful array of fruits to your dish of quinoa or oats. Antioxidants like anthocyanins and flavonoids, which are abundant in berries like strawberries, blueberries, and raspberries, have been demonstrated to prevent heart disease by lowering inflammation and enhancing blood vessel function. A ripe banana adds potassium, which is a mineral that supports the health of the heart muscle and helps control blood pressure.

As you proceed to construct your breakfast masterpiece, remember to include sources of good fats. A small handful of nuts or seeds, like almonds, walnuts, or chia seeds, can be added to food to increase the amount of heart-healthy monounsaturated and polyunsaturated fats and omega-3 fatty acids, which can lower blood triglyceride levels and lower the risk of arrhythmias. You can get extra monounsaturated fats, potassium, and fiber by slicing up some creamy avocado.

In order to complete your breakfast, think about including a source of lean protein. Eggs are a flexible choice that supply important minerals like vitamin D and choline as well as high-quality protein. Choosing Greek yogurt also provides probiotics, which can help lower inflammation and improve gastrointestinal health, both of which may be beneficial to heart health. You may add protein to your breakfast without consuming too much saturated fat by providing lean meats like grilled chicken sausage or turkey bacon.

To accompany your heart-healthy breakfast, don't forget to hydrate with a glass of water or a cup of green tea. Staying hydrated is essential for maintaining proper blood flow and supporting overall heart function. Green tea contains catechins, powerful antioxidants that have been linked to reduced risk of heart disease and stroke.

By starting your day with a breakfast that nourishes your body and supports your heart health, you're setting yourself up for a day of vitality and well-being. So go ahead, savor each bite of your breakfast delight, knowing that you're taking a proactive step towards a healthier heart.

Energizing Smoothie Bowls

Making nutritious smoothie bowls that are full of heart-healthy ingredients is a fun project for the kitchen. These colorful mixtures not only entice the palate but also strengthen the heart, guaranteeing a harmonious blend of well-being with every bite.

Begin by assembling a kaleidoscope of fresh, organic fruits such as succulent berries, luscious mangoes, and creamy avocado, all teeming with antioxidants that shield the heart from oxidative stress. These jewel-toned gems not only impart a burst of flavor but also bestow a plethora of vitamins and minerals essential for cardiovascular vitality

Next, introduce a symphony of wholesome seeds and nuts, such as chia seeds, flaxseeds, and almonds, to infuse the smoothie bowl with a potent dose of omega-3 fatty acids and plant-based protein. These nutrient powerhouses work synergistically to regulate cholesterol levels and promote optimal heart function, elevating the bowl from a mere culinary delight to a heart-healthy masterpiece.

To amplify the nutritional prowess of the smoothie bowl, incorporate vibrant greens like spinach and kale, verdant superfoods renowned for their abundance of folate, potassium, and fiber. These verdant wonders not only lend a verdant hue to the bowl but also bolster cardiovascular health by reducing inflammation and supporting healthy blood pressure levels.

For a creamy indulgence sans guilt, opt for a velvety base of Greek yogurt or coconut milk, brimming with probiotics and medium-chain triglycerides that nourish the gut microbiome and foster overall cardiovascular wellness. This creamy canvas serves as the perfect backdrop for the vibrant medley of fruits, seeds, and greens, harmonizing flavors and textures in a symphony of healthful decadence.

Add toasted coconut flakes, crunchy granola clusters, and a drizzle of raw honey or pure maple syrup for a hint of natural sweetness to the smoothie bowl to enhance the flavor experience. These mouthwatering toppings give the bowl an enticing charm and a lovely crunch that invites the palette to relish each mouthful to the fullest.
energizing smoothie bowls for heart health are not merely culinary creations but culinary works of art, meticulously crafted to nourish the body and delight the senses. With a harmonious blend of vibrant fruits, wholesome seeds, verdant greens, and creamy indulgences, these bowls offer a symphony of flavor and nutrition that invigorates the heart and soul with every luscious bite.

Wholesome Oatmeal Varieties

Oatmeal, a venerable grain with a rich history dating back millennia, stands as a cornerstone in the realm of heart-healthy cuisine. Its versatility knows no bounds, offering a canvas upon which culinary creativity flourishes. Within the spectrum of wholesome oatmeal varieties lie a plethora of options, each brimming with unique flavors, textures, and nutritional benefits, tailor-made to support cardiovascular wellness.

Let us embark on a gastronomic journey, exploring the multifaceted world of heart-healthy oatmeal recipes:

Steel-Cut Oats: Steel-cut oats, the unwavering defender of healthful grains, will take you on a trip through the ages. Scooped from the groat's inner kernel, these oats have a strong, nutty flavor and a chewy texture that leaves a satisfying mouthfeel. Steel-cut oats, which are high in soluble fiber, lower cholesterol and increase fullness, making them a heart-healthy star.

Rolled Oats: Enter the realm of familiarity with rolled oats, beloved for their convenience and versatility. These oats, gently flattened through the rolling process, offer a tender, creamy consistency that lends itself beautifully to a myriad of culinary endeavors. Packed with fiber and nutrients, rolled oats serve as a steadfast ally in the quest for heart health, bestowing upon the discerning palate a symphony of wholesome goodness.

Oat Groats: The raw diamonds of the oat world, oat groats will transport you to a world of rustic beauty. Renowned for their robust texture and earthy taste, these whole grains are a tribute to the unadulterated abundance of nature. With every delicious spoonful, oat groats, bursting with vital nutrients and fiber, constitute a genuine powerhouse of cardiovascular support, strengthening the body and feeding the soul.

Oat Bran: The nutrient-rich outer layer of the oat kernel, oat bran will take you on a gourmet journey of discovery. Packed with fiber and antioxidants, this little yet powerful ingredient is a mainstay of heart-healthy cooking. A diet rich in advantages can be achieved by including oat bran, which also pleases the palate with its mild, nutty flavor. Other benefits include blood sugar stabilization and digestive health promotion.

Multigrain Oatmeal: A delicious medley of oats and other healthful grains, multigrain oatmeal is a great way to start an epicurean exploration. Culinary fusion talent is demonstrated by this harmonious blend of flavors and textures, skillfully crafted to entice the senses and provide nourishment for the body. Multigrain oatmeal, full of fiber, vitamins, and minerals, is a sensory overload that provides a harmonious blend of healthful deliciousness with each bite.

There is a large and abundant universe of heart-healthy oatmeal variations available for recipes, just waiting for investigation and creative cooking. There are many variations to satisfy every taste and inclination, whether one favors the hearty charm of steel-cut oats or the cozy embrace of rolled oats. Through the consumption of these nutritious grains, one can take a step toward the best possible cardiovascular health and enjoy every mouthful along the way.

Nutrient-packed Breakfast Muffins

These hearty muffins are a great way to start the day because they are packed with nutrients that will power your body and heart. Not only are these muffins delicious, but they also improve your overall health because they are loaded with heart-healthy components and vital nutrients. Come with me as we explore the components and advantages of this wholesome dish.

Ingredients:

Whole Grain Flour: To increase dietary fiber and encourage heart health, use whole grain flour rather than processed flour.

Oats: Packed with soluble fiber, oats reduce blood sugar swings and cholesterol while promoting cardiovascular health.

Omega-3 fatty acids found in flaxseeds help to lower cholesterol and reduce inflammation, which is why flax seeds are good for heart health.

Protein and microorganisms found in **Greek yogurt** help to maintain gastrointestinal health and improve cardiovascular function in general.

Berries: Brimming with vitamins and antioxidants, berries minimize the risk of heart disease by battling inflammation and oxidative stress.

Nuts: Pecans, walnuts, or almonds give the muffins crunch and heart-healthy fats that support cardiovascular health.

Bananas: Known for their natural sweetness and high potassium content, bananas promote heart health and blood pressure regulation.

Honey: Adding sweetness without dramatically raising blood sugar levels, honey is a natural sweetener with antioxidant qualities.

Instructions:

Adjust the oven temperature to 350°F (175°C) and grease or line a muffin tray.

Combine whole grain flour, ground flaxseeds, oats, and your preferred nuts in a big bowl.

Mash ripe bananas and mix with Greek yogurt and honey in a different bowl.

Stirring until just blended, gradually add the wet components to the dry ingredients.

Add your preferred frozen or fresh berries and fold gently.

Pour the batter into each muffin tin, filling it to about three-quarters of the way to the top.

When a toothpick is placed into the center, the baked food should come out clean after 20 to 25 minutes.

Before putting the muffins on a wire rack to cool entirely, let them cool for a few minutes.

Benefits:

Heart Health: Fiber, omega-3 fatty acids, antioxidants, potassium, and a variety of other nutrients are found in whole grains, oats, flaxseeds, nuts, and berries. These nutrients also reinforce heart health.

Insulin resistance and type 2 diabetes are less likely to occur thanks to the blood sugar-regulating properties of the fiber-rich components in these muffins.

gut health: Greek yogurt contains probiotics that help maintain a balanced gut microbiota and, by enhancing nutrient absorption and digestion, may lower the risk of heart disease.

Antioxidant Protection: Rich sources of antioxidants, such as berries and honey, help fend against oxidative stress and inflammation, two major causes of heart disease.

Satiety and Weight Management: These muffins' protein, fiber, and healthy fats all work together to enhance satiety, which reduces cravings and supports weight management—a crucial aspect of heart health. 25

These heart-healthy, tasty, and portable breakfast muffins are a great way to start your day. They are high in nutrients. You can eat a diet rich in whole grains, oats, flaxseeds, almonds, berries, and other nutritious foods to support cardiovascular health. Savor these muffins as part of a well-rounded diet, and take pride in your proactive efforts to maintain a healthier heart.

Chapter 2 Light and Flavorful Starters

Here's a thorough explanation of heart-healthy, tasty, and light starters:

Crispy Citrus Salad with Shrimp and Avocado

This colorful appetizer pairs creamy avocado with juicy shrimp and the crisp tang of citrus fruits. To start, put together a mixture of fresh citrus fruits, like oranges, grapefruits, and tangerines. Remove the seeds and pitch before slicing them into segments. Next, carefully combine fried shrimp and diced ripe avocado with the citrus segments. Add some finely chopped fresh herbs, such mint or cilantro, for texture and taste.

While the avocado adds heart-healthy monounsaturated fats, the citrus fruits in this salad give a dose of vitamin C. This appetizer is filling and nutrient-dense because shrimp is a lean source of protein. The dish is light and refreshing, making it the ideal way to start a heart-healthy meal. The combination of flavors and textures.

Platter of Grilled Vegetable Antipasto

A variety of flavor-bursting grilled vegetables are included on this vibrant antipasto plate. Choose a range of seasonal veggies to start, like bell peppers, zucchini, eggplant, and asparagus. Cut the veggies into uniform-sized pieces and give them a quick olive oil brushing. Add a dash of pepper, salt, and your preferred herbs and spices for seasoning. After the vegetables are soft and gently browned from the grill, place them on a dish.

With their abundance of vitamins, minerals, and antioxidants, the grilled veggies on this antipasto platter are a great option for heart health. The recipe gains depth from the smoky taste that the grilling method imparts, allowing the naturally sweet veggies to take center stage. To boost the protein and taste of the platter, serve it over a serving of baba ganoush or hummus.

Salad of fresh herbs and poached salmon

A vivid salsa created with fresh herbs and lemon atop delicate poached salmon, this is a sophisticated appetizer. Salmon filets should first be gently poached in a solution of water, white wine, and aromatics like lemon segments, peppercorns, and fresh herbs. Transfer the salmon gently to a serving tray once it's flaky and cooked through.

Finely chop a variety of fresh herbs, including parsley, dill, chives, and basil, to make the herb salsa. Add the chopped tomatoes, garlic, shallots, and herbs to a bowl and toss. After adding salt and pepper to taste, generously spread the salsa over the poached salmon.

Omega-3 fatty acids, which are abundant in salmon, have been demonstrated to promote heart health by lowering cholesterol and reducing inflammation. In addition to adding taste and brightness to the dish, the fresh herb salsa also provides extra minerals and antioxidants. This sophisticated appetizer will warm the hearts of your visitors while making a lasting impression.

These appetizers are rich in nutrients that promote heart health in addition to being tasty and filling. These recipes offer a tasty way to start a heart-healthy dinner by combining a range of fresh ingredients, such as citrus fruits, vegetables, and lean proteins.

Fresh Salad Creations

Start by choosing a range of nutrient-rich ingredients recognized for their cardiovascular advantages while crafting heart-healthy meals at Fresh Salad Creations. Following is a detailed how-to:

Leafy Greens: Start with a bed of leafy greens, like arugula, spinach, or kale. These leafy vegetables are rich in antioxidants, minerals, and vitamins that promote heart health.

Lean Proteins: Include grilled chicken, tofu, or chickpeas in your salad as a source of lean protein. These proteins support heart health by supplying necessary amino acids without an excessive amount of saturated fat.

Vibrant Fruits and Vegetables: Add a range of vibrant fruits and vegetables, such as citrus segments, bell peppers, cucumbers, and berries. These colorful garnishes not only make your salad look better, but they also contribute a variety of heart-healthy elements.

Add sources of heart-healthy fats, like almonds or avocado, to your diet. Both avocado and nuts offer a wealth of monounsaturated fats and omega-3 fatty acids, which have been demonstrated to promote cardiovascular health.

Whole Grains: To get an additional boost of fiber and complex carbohydrates, try mixing in whole grains such as brown rice or quinoa to your salad. These grains support heart health by promoting satiety and stabilizing blood sugar levels.

Make Your Own Dressings: Incorporate heart-healthy oils such as olive oil into your homemade dressings, along with aromatic herbs and spices. Use natural substances to improve flavor without sacrificing health, rather than adding too much sugar or salt.

Portion Control: To guarantee a well-balanced meal, pay attention to portion quantities. Salads are healthful, but eating too much of anything, even good food, can result in consuming too many calories, which over time can affect heart health.

With these simple steps and an assortment of heart-healthy ingredients, you can make delectable, heart-healthy recipes at Fresh Salad Creations that satisfy the body and the spirit.

Hearty Vegetable Soups

Filling and Heart-Healthy Vegetable Soup: A Glass of Well-Being

Overview: This recipe for Hearty Vegetable Soup is a carefully prepared step toward heart health through food. This soup is a symphony of sustenance and wellness, full of colorful, nutrient-dense veggies and tastes that dance beautifully on the palate.

Ingredients list:

Two teaspoons of olive oil

Finely slice one big onion.

Diced one red bell pepper, chopped one zucchini, minced two carrots, diced two celery stalks, diced one cup green beans, cut and trimmed

Chopped tomatoes (fresh or canned) in one cup

Four cups of veggie broth with minimal sodium

One tsp. of dried thyme

one tsp of dried rosemary

Add salt and black pepper to taste.

- For garnish, use fresh parsley.

Guidelines:

Sauteing Symphony: Set a big pot over medium heat to begin orchestrating the sautéing process. Add the minced garlic and finely sliced onions, and let them serenade one another until fragrant and tender.

Vegetable Crescendo: Add the chopped celery, red bell pepper, zucchini, green beans, and carrots to the pot and allow them to blend in with the other flavors in a harmonious ensemble. Stirring from time to time allows the vegetables to release their aromatic essence as they dance and interact.

Harmonious Infusion: Add a pinch of dried thyme and rosemary to the pot and let their earthy undertones combine with the veggies, producing a flavorful symphony. To enhance the depth of flavor, season with a touch of salt and a good crush of black pepper.

Broth Overture: Cover the vegetables with a warm, soothing layer of low-sodium vegetable broth by pouring it into the saucepan. Let the soup simmer gently so that the ingredients can combine and harmonize, producing a mouthwatering song of flavor.

Simmering Serenity: Let the soup simmer gently for 20-25 minutes, allowing the vegetables to reach a state of tender perfection while the broth becomes imbued with their essence. Taste and adjust seasoning if necessary, ensuring a perfectly balanced flavor profile.

Finale Flourish: Serve the Hearty Vegetable Soup hot, garnished with freshly chopped parsley, a verdant flourish that adds a final touch of freshness and vibrancy to this nourishing masterpiece.

Advantages:

Savor this harmonious blend of flavors for its many health advantages in addition to its delicious flavor. Brimming with antioxidants, vitamins, and fiber, this heart-healthy vegetable soup satisfies the body and spirit while fostering general health and vigor. Enjoy the culinary genius and relish every morsel of goodness, knowing that you are nourishing your body and soul with every mouthful.

Tasty Hummus and Veggie Dips

Gather the following ingredients to make a heart-healthy hummus and veggie dip: olive oil, lemon juice, garlic, tahini, chickpeas, and a variety of fresh vegetables–carrots, cucumbers, bell peppers, and celery–for dipping.

A can of chickpeas should be rinsed and drained before being added to a food processor.

Add the two tablespoons of tahini, one lemon's juice, two chopped garlic cloves, and two teaspoons of olive oil to the food processor with the chickpeas.

Using a spatula if needed, blend the ingredients until they are smooth.

One tablespoon of water at a time can be added to the hummus if it's too thick until the right consistency is achieved.

After tasting the hummus, taste and adjust the seasoning with more salt and pepper if necessary.

Before serving, move the hummus onto a bowl and pour in a little additional olive oil.

Regarding the vegetable dip:

Pick a range of fresh veggies, including celery, bell peppers, cucumbers, and carrots.

Clean the veggies and cut them into little pieces.

Arrange the veggies around the hummus dish on a serving tray.

For appearance and taste enhancement, you can optionally top the hummus and veggies with some finely chopped fresh herbs.

This hummus and veggie dip is a heart-healthy snack or appetizer because it's full of fiber, vitamins, and minerals. Olive oil contributes healthful lipids, and chickpeas offer fiber and plant-based protein. The fresh veggies make a great dip because they're full of nutrients and low in calories. Savor this tasty and wholesome snack whenever you want!

Chapter 3 Nourishing Main Courses

Of course! The following heart-healthy recipes for nutritious main courses:

To make Grilled Salmon with Herb Crust, first marinate fresh salmon filets in a solution of lemon juice, olive oil, and minced garlic.

Grate some lemon zest and mix in some finely chopped parsley and dill to make a herb crust.

Once the fish is fully cooked and the herb crust is aromatic and golden, grill it.

Accompany with a colorful mixed green salad with avocado, cherry tomatoes, and a mild vinaigrette.

Bell peppers stuffed with quinoa:

Prepare the quinoa as directed on the package and combine it with the corn, black beans, chopped tomatoes, onions, and garlic that have been sautéed.

Remove the seeds and membranes from bell peppers by cutting them in half, then stuff the peppers with the quinoa mixture.

Bake until the filling is thoroughly cooked and the peppers are soft.

Before serving, put some finely grated low-fat cheese and chopped fresh cilantro on top.

Roasted vegetables and chicken with lemon herbs:

Marinate skinless, boneless chicken breasts in a concoction of fresh herbs such as oregano, rosemary, and thyme, together with lemon juice and olive oil.

Bake the chicken in the oven until it is well done and nicely browned.

In the meantime, roast a variety of bright veggies, including bell peppers, carrots, and Brussels sprouts, with the chicken until they are soft. Toss them with olive oil, salt, and pepper.

For a filling supper, serve the chicken and roasted veggies with brown rice or whole grain couscous on the side.

Curry with Lentils and Veggies:

Fry the ginger, garlic, and onions in a big pot until aromatic. Add the zucchini, bell peppers, and sliced carrots.

Stir in the cooked lentils, canned diced tomatoes, vegetable broth, and a blend of curry powders (turmeric, cumin, and coriander).

Simmer the vegetables until they are tender and the flavors have blended.

Serve the curry over brown rice or cooked quinoa, garnished with chopped fresh cilantro and a dollop of Greek yogurt for added richness.

Not only are these heart-healthy main dishes delightful, but they are also nutrient-rich and enhance general well-being.

Lean Protein Entrées

Colorful Veggie Stir-Fries

Not only are colorful veggie stir-fries and lean protein entrées delightful, but they are also vital parts of a heart-healthy diet. Including lean proteins in your diet, such as those found in fish, poultry, tofu, or lentils, gives your body the essential nutrients it needs—like zinc, iron, and protein—without adding too much saturated fat, which raises the risk of heart disease. Additionally, these proteins lessen the chance of overeating by keeping you feeling content and full.

The range of veggies used in colorful veggie stir-fries not only adds a plethora of vitamins, minerals, and antioxidants to your meal, but also brilliant hues. Rich in fiber, vitamins A and C, potassium, and folate, vegetables such as bell peppers, broccoli, carrots, and spinach are also high in these nutrients, which are vital for heart health. The vibrant variety of veggies also offers phytonutrients, which have been connected to lowering the risk of heart disease and inflammation.

Stir-frying colorful vegetables with lean proteins results in well-balanced meals that are not only heart-healthy but also palatable. Food is swiftly cooked at high heat when stir-fried, preserving the nutrients in the components. You may increase the health advantages of these dishes even further by using less oil and flavoring them with herbs and spices in place of salt.

Start with selecting your protein source and cooking it in a healthy way to make a lean protein entrée with a vibrant veggie stir-fry. For instance, before grilling or baking, you can marinate chicken breast in a solution of lemon juice, garlic, and herbs. As an alternative, you can pan-sear tofu and give it a thin layer of cornstarch to make it crispy.

While your protein is cooking, chop a variety of vibrant veggies, like snap peas, mushrooms, zucchini, and red and yellow bell peppers. Start with the vegetables that take longer to cook and add them in batches to a wok or big pan that has been heated with a tiny amount of oil over medium-high heat. Once the vegetables are crisp-tender, add the cooked protein to the skillet and stir-fry it for a few minutes.

Add some garlic, ginger, chili flakes, low-sodium soy sauce, or tamari to your stir-fry to give it flavor without using too much salt or sweet sauces. To develop distinctive flavor profiles, try experimenting with additional seasonings like curry powder, cumin, or sesame oil.

After everything is done, enjoy a filling and nutritious supper by serving your colorful veggie stir-fry and lean protein entrée over cooked brown rice, quinoa, or cauliflower rice. Along with providing your body with heart-healthy nutrients, you'll also be indulging your taste buds with a delectable culinary experience that's as pleasurable as it is healthful.

Balanced Grain Bowls

Okay, let's get started on making a heart-healthy, well-balanced grain bowl that tastes great.
First, choose a whole grain basis (quinoa, brown rice, or farro are good options). The minerals and fiber in these grains help to maintain heart health. Grain should be cooked as directed on the bag until it's soft but still somewhat chewy.

Then fill your bowl with an assortment of vibrant veggies. Include colorful vegetables such as bell peppers, carrots, and cherry tomatoes, and choose leafy greens like spinach or kale. These veggies are a great source of vitamins and antioxidants that support heart health.

Add lean protein sources like beans, tofu, or grilled chicken breast. In addition to promoting muscle health, protein keeps you feeling full and content. Instead of using salt to season your protein, use herbs and spices to lower your intake of sodium.

Add foods like avocado slices, almonds, or seeds to your bowl to add healthy fats. These fats have the ability to cut cholesterol and lower the risk of heart disease. In addition, they give your dish a delightfully creamy and crunchy texture.

Pour a homemade vinaigrette, composed of heart-healthy olive oil, lemon juice, and herbs, over your grain bowl at the end. This dressing gives taste without being overly heavy in fat or sodium.

Arrange your veggies, protein, and healthy fats on top of a base of cooked grains. Finally, top with freshly grated Parmesan cheese or fresh herbs, if preferred. Drizzle with the prepared vinaigrette.

Savor the heart-healthy benefits of your balanced grain bowl as a filling and nutritious lunch!

Chapter 4 Satisfying Sides and Snacks

Adding filling sides and snacks to your diet is a great way to enjoy tasty flavors without sacrificing heart health. Imagine bright, vibrant salads with an abundance of fresh vegetables mixed with a zesty vinaigrette. Or how about some roasted sweet potatoes that have been seasoned with a dash of savory herbs to give them a delightful crunch with every bite? If you're looking for heart-healthy fats and protein to keep you feeling full and energized throughout the day, try crunchy nuts and seeds.

Not to be overlooked is the ageless classic of crunchy, crisp vegetables and creamy hummus combined for a filling and healthy snack. These options enhance cardiovascular health by contributing to a balanced diet while also tantalizing the taste sensations.

Oven-Baked Sweet Potato Fries

Here's a quick and heart-healthy recipe for oven-baked sweet potato fries:

Ingredients:

Two substantial sweet potatoes

Two tsp olive oil

One tsp of paprika

one tsp powdered garlic

One tsp powdered onion

To taste, add salt and pepper.

Instructions:

Turn the oven on to 425°F (220°C).

Assemble the sweet potatoes. After carefully cleaning, peel the sweet potatoes. Slice them into slender, 1/4-inch-thick pieces.

Garnish the fries: Combine the olive oil, paprika, onion, garlic, and pepper powders with the sweet potato strips in a big bowl and toss until well coated.

Place on a baking sheet. Aluminum foil or parchment paper can be used to line a baking pan. Don't overcrowd the baking pan; instead, arrange the seasoned sweet potato fries in a single layer. Their consistent crisping is made possible by this.

Bake: After preheating the oven, place the baking sheet inside and bake the fries for 25 to 30 minutes, turning them over halfway through, or until they are crispy and golden brown.

Serve: Take the baked sweet potato fries out of the oven and allow them to cool for a few minutes before cutting into serving size portions. Savor them as a tasty and nutritious snack or side dish!

Time Spent Preparing: about fifteen minutes
Cook for 25 to 30 minutes.

These oven-baked sweet potato fries are not only delicious but also heart-healthy, providing plenty of vitamins and minerals without the excess fat and calories of traditional fries.

Crunchy Kale Chips

To make crispy, heart-healthy kale chips, follow these instructions:
Set oven temperature to 300°F, or 150°C.

Using a kitchen towel or salad spinner, carefully wash and pat dry the kale leaves.

Tear the kale leaves into bite-sized pieces after removing the stiff stems.

Lightly cover the kale pieces with a little amount of olive oil by tossing them in a big basin. For even covering, work the oil into the leaves.

Use your preferred spices or seasonings to season the greens. For a cheesy flavor, popular choices include sea salt, black pepper, garlic powder, or nutritional yeast.

Arrange the seasoned kale pieces in a single layer on a baking sheet that has silicone baking mats or parchment paper on it. To guarantee crispiness, make sure there aren't too many of them.

For around 15 to 20 minutes, or until they are crispy but not burnt, bake the kale chips in a preheated oven. Watch them closely because they can turn from crispy to burnt very fast.

When finished, take the kale chips out of the oven and allow them to cool a little before serving. Savor your heart-healthy crunchy kale chips as a wholesome after-meal snack or as an appetizer.

Protein-Packed Snack

To craft Protein-Packed Snack Bites as part of a heart-healthy recipe, you'll need a solid foundation of protein-rich ingredients like nuts, seeds, or nut butter. These elements not only provide essential protein but also healthy fats and fiber, contributing to heart health. Begin by selecting a base such as almonds, walnuts, or a combination of both, as they contain heart-healthy fats and provide a satisfying crunch.

Add in seeds such as hemp, flax, or chia seeds next. Packed with fiber, protein, and omega-3 fatty acids, these little powerhouses promote heart health. They also have a pleasing texture that can help you feel content and full for longer.

Use natural sweeteners, such as dates, honey, or maple syrup, to enhance flavor and sweetness without using processed sugars. Dates give the snack bits their chewy texture in addition to adding sweetness. They also include a lot of potassium, which helps to regulate blood pressure and heart health.

If you want to further improve the nutritional profile, you might add superfoods like cacao powder or nibs. Antioxidants found in cacao, especially flavonoids, have been related to heart health advantages like lowered blood pressure and better blood flow.

Finally, to aid in keeping the components together, think about adding a binding agent like coconut oil or nut butter. Nut butter increases protein and good fats while adding richness and creaminess. In addition to providing medium-chain triglycerides (MCTs), which have been linked to better heart health, coconut oil can also help create a smooth texture.

After gathering all of your ingredients, put them in a food processor and pulse until a smooth consistency forms. After that, shape the dough into bite-sized balls and place them in the refrigerator to firm up for at least half an hour.

In addition to being tasty, these protein-packed snack bites are a handy and wholesome way to satiate hunger in between meals and promote heart health. Moreover, you can experiment with different nuts, seeds, and flavorings to fit your taste preferences because they are adjustable.

Chapter 5 Sweet Treats with a Healthy Twist

"Delicious Treats with a Heart-Healthy Perspective: Creating Sweet Concoctions with a Nutritious Aspect"

Introduction:

Eating delicious desserts doesn't have to conflict with leading a heart-healthy lifestyle. Accept the challenge of creating delicious treats with a healthy twist so that every mouthful not only satisfies the palate but also provides nourishment for the body. With these creative recipes that balance flavor, health, and satisfaction, you can take your cooking to the next level.

Section 1: Enlightening Ingredients

Embark on a culinary odyssey with a curated selection of wholesome ingredients, meticulously chosen to infuse each creation with goodness. Harness the power of nature's bounty, incorporating nutrient-rich elements such as antioxidant-laden berries, heart-friendly nuts, and wholesome whole grains.

Discover the magic of ingredient synergy, where tastes and textures blend together to create a satisfying symphony without sacrificing health. Use natural sweeteners instead of refined sugars to enhance your recipes, such as pure maple syrup and honey.

Section 2: Crafting Confections with Care

As you begin the adventure of creating confections with painstaking attention to detail and care, you will enter the realm of culinary artistry. Accept cutting-edge methods and gastronomic knowledge to elevate basic materials into exquisite works of art that satiate the senses.

Discover how to create a harmonious blend of crisp freshness, creamy pleasure, and subtle sweetness in a delectable richness. Let every dish you make serve as a tribute to the union of exquisite taste and healthful ingredients.

Section 3: Divine Desserts, Heart-Healthy Pleasures

Discover a plethora of mouth watering sweets that have been redesigned with heart health in mind. Each creation offers a guilt-free treat that nourishes both body and soul, from rich almond flour brownies to velvety chocolate avocado mousse.

Savor every delicious taste with the peace of mind that comes from knowing that every morsel was created with intention and care. Let these confections serve as a celebration of life, love, and the skill of providing oneself with healthful, delicious food.

Savor every delicious meal with the knowledge that every piece is expertly made, and revel in the delight of guilt-free indulgence. Let these desserts serve as a celebration of life, love, and the skill of feeding oneself well.

Fruit-Filled Dessert Parfaits

Here's a novel approach to creating heart-healthy fruit-filled dessert parfaits:

Choose a range of fresh fruits to start, such as pineapple, kiwi, mango, and berries. These fruits are a heart-healthy source of vitamins, minerals, and antioxidants.
Peel and cut the fruits into small pieces. Ensure that all seeds and pits are eliminated.
Next, use low-fat or Greek yogurt to prepare a heart-healthy concoction. Yogurt's probiotics reduce

inflammation and raise cholesterol, which is beneficial to heart health.

In parfait glasses or bowls, arrange the yogurt and chopped fruits in layers. Yogurt should be layered first, then mixed fruits should come next. Continue doing this until the glass is full, then top it off with a dollop of yogurt.

Top the parfait with some heart-healthy toppings, such granola or chopped nuts, for some extra crunchy and taste. Nuts are high in fiber, plant sterols, and unsaturated fats that can help lower cholesterol and lower the risk of heart disease.

If you'd like, drizzle a little honey or maple syrup over the parfait to add a little sweetness. Remember to use these sweeteners sparingly in order to preserve a balance that is heart-healthy.

Finally, for an added flavor and antioxidant boost, top the parfait with a sprinkling of cinnamon or a sprig of fresh mint.

Savor your wholesome and delectable Fruit-Filled Dessert Parfait as a heart-healthy and fulfilling dessert!

Guilt-Free Dark Chocolate Treats

Combining wholesome components with cocoa's richness allows for the creation of guilt-free, heart-healthy dark chocolate desserts. Start by finding premium dark chocolate that has at least 70% cocoa content. Next, enhance its health advantages by adding organic sweeteners like honey or maple syrup—avoid processed sweets. Increase the nutritional value by adding healthy ingredients such as nuts, seeds, or dried fruit to give it a nice crunch and a boost of fiber.

To improve the creamy texture and support heart health, use unsaturated fats like avocado or coconut oil. Lastly, to enhance the chocolatey flavor and achieve a balanced taste, add a small amount of sea salt. Savor these treats without feeling guilty as a delicious complement to your heart-healthy lifestyle.

Baked Fruit Crisps

Ingredients: Whole wheat flour, eggs, low-fat milk, honey, mixed berries (such as strawberries, blueberries, and raspberries), and a pinch of cinnamon.

Batter Preparation: In a mixing bowl, combine 1 cup of whole wheat flour, 2 eggs, 1 cup of low-fat milk, and 1 tablespoon of honey. Whisk until smooth.

Preheat Oven: Preheat your oven to 350°F (175°C).

Fruit Filling: Wash and slice the mixed berries. Toss them with a sprinkle of cinnamon.

Baking: Lightly grease a baking dish. Pour a thin layer of the batter into the dish. Arrange the mixed berries over the batter. Pour the remaining batter over the berries.

Bake: After the oven has been prepared, put the baking dish in and bake for 20 to 25 minutes, or until the center is set and the rims are golden brown.

Serving: Allow the crepes to cool slightly after baking before slicing and serving. Take pleasure in your heart-healthy baked fruit crepes!

Explanation:

Whole Wheat Flour: Provides fiber which is good for heart health.

Eggs: A source of protein which is important for muscle and heart health.

Low-fat Milk: Contains calcium and protein with less saturated fat than whole milk.

Honey: Adds natural sweetness without refined sugars.

Mixed Berries: Packed with antioxidants and fiber, beneficial for heart health.

Cinnamon: Adds flavor without the need for excess sugar and has potential heart health benefits.

Chapter 6 Meal Planning and Success Strategies

For the purpose of keeping a balanced diet and preserving time and money, meal planning is essential. Here are a few successful strategies:

Establish Realistic Goals: Assess your nutritional requirements, tastes, and objectives (e.g., to lose weight, increase muscle, or just eat a healthy diet).

Make a Plan: Every week, set aside time to prepare your meals. Take into account elements like your family's tastes, schedule, and ingredients that are on hand.

Establish a Menu: Provide a range of well-balanced meals, such as lean proteins, whole grains, fruits, and vegetables, on a weekly or monthly basis.

Cooking in batches: Make big quantities of basic items, such as cereals, proteins, and sauces, in advance to use over the week.

Use Leftovers: Repurpose leftovers into new meals to minimize food waste and save time.

Shop Smart: Make a shopping list based on your meal plan to avoid impulse buys and ensure you have all the necessary ingredients.

Stay Flexible: Be open to making adjustments based on changes in your schedule, cravings, or ingredient availability.

Portion Control: Practice portion control to avoid overeating and ensure you're getting the right balance of nutrients.

Stay Organized: Keep your kitchen organized and stocked with healthy options to make meal preparation easier.

Track Your Progress: Keep an eye on your meals and make necessary adjustments to your plan to make sure you're sticking to your nutrition schedule and reaching your goals.

Track your progress with this bonus time table

Day	Recipes	Date

Conclusion: Embracing a Heart-Healthy Lifestyle

As we conclude this culinary exploration of heart health, let's celebrate the achievement of our efforts. These meals have been a symphony of flavors and a mosaic of nutrients that have not only fueled our bodies but also lifted our moods. As we say goodbye to our culinary journey, let's continue the tradition of healthful eating and foster a positive connection between our hearts and our palates. Cheers to many more culinary explorations,

where each dish serves as a symbol of our dedication to
overall health.